THE DYSPHAGIA DIET BIBLE

Beginners Practical Dietary Guidance For Dysphagia & Recipes And Tips For Safe Eating

CRUE GAGE

Table of Contents

Introductory

Dysphagia is a medical term that refers to the inability to ingest. A multitude of factors can contribute to its occurrence, including neurological conditions (such as Parkinson's disease or stroke), structural issues (such as strictures or tumors), or muscular disorders.

Symptoms may encompass the sensation of food becoming lodged in the esophagus or chest, coughing or choking during meals, or experiencing discomfort while swallowing. The treatment is contingent upon the underlying cause and may involve dietary modifications, dysphagia therapy, or medical interventions.

Causes And Types

Dysphagia can be classified into two main types based on the phase of swallowing affected:

• **Oropharyngeal Dysphagia**: Difficulty initiating the swallowing process, often involving the mouth and throat. Causes can include:

1. Neurological disorders (e.g., stroke, Parkinson's disease, multiple sclerosis)
2. Muscular disorders (e.g., muscular dystrophy)
3. Structural abnormalities (e.g., tumors, inflammation)

• **Esophageal Dysphagia**: Difficulty moving food down the esophagus. Causes can include:

- Esophageal strictures (narrowing of the esophagus)
- Achalasia (a condition affecting the muscles of the esophagus)
- Gastroesophageal reflux disease (GERD)
- Tumors or other obstructions

<u>Other causes may include:</u>

- Aging
- Infections
- Medications that affect swallowing or esophageal motility
- Inflammatory conditions (e.g., eosinophilic esophagitis)

Understanding the specific type and cause of dysphagia is crucial for effective treatment.

<u>**Diet management is crucial for individuals with dysphagia for several reasons:**</u>

• **Safety**: Proper dietary modifications can help prevent choking or aspiration (food entering the airway), which can lead to pneumonia or other serious complications.

• **Nutritional Adequacy**: Adapting the diet ensures that individuals receive the necessary nutrients, as swallowing difficulties may limit food choices.

• **Improved Quality of Life**: A well-managed diet can enhance the enjoyment of meals and social interactions, reducing the stress associated with eating.

• **Swallowing Efficiency**: Certain food textures (e.g., pureed or thickened liquids) can make swallowing easier and more effective, minimizing discomfort and improving swallowing function.

• **Preventing Malnutrition and Dehydration**: Careful dietary planning helps avoid malnutrition and dehydration, which are common risks for individuals with dysphagia.

Overall, diet management tailored to the individual's specific needs is an essential component of dysphagia treatment and care.

CHAPTER ONE
Assessment Of Dysphagia

The assessment of dysphagia typically involves several steps to determine the cause and severity of the condition. Here are the key components:

- **Clinical Evaluation**: A healthcare provider conducts a thorough medical history and physical examination. This includes discussing symptoms, duration, and any associated issues (like weight loss or coughing during meals).

- **Swallowing Assessment**: A bedside swallowing assessment may be performed, where the patient swallows various food textures and liquids under observation. This helps identify specific difficulties.

- **Modified Barium Swallow Study (MBSS)**: This X-ray test evaluates swallowing function in real-time as the patient consumes food mixed with barium. It helps visualize the swallowing process and identify abnormalities.

- **Fiberoptic Endoscopic Evaluation of Swallowing (FEES)**: This involves inserting a flexible endoscope through the nose to observe the throat and swallowing function directly. It can assess the safety and efficiency of swallowing.

- **Manometry**: This test measures the pressure and function of the esophagus, helping diagnose motility disorders that may cause dysphagia.

- **Nutritional Assessment**: Evaluating dietary intake and nutritional status to identify any deficiencies that may arise due to swallowing difficulties.

The results from these assessments guide treatment planning and dietary modifications to ensure safety and nutritional adequacy.

Nutritional Considerations

Nutritional considerations for individuals with dysphagia are essential to ensure they receive adequate nutrition while maintaining safety during eating and drinking. Here are key points to consider:

• **Texture Modifications**: Foods and liquids may need to be modified to facilitate safe swallowing. This often involves altering textures, such as pureeing foods, thickening liquids, or using soft, moist foods that are easier to swallow.

- **Balanced Diet**: Despite texture modifications, it's crucial to maintain a balanced diet that includes a variety of nutrients. This can be achieved through specialized products or recipes designed for dysphagia, which ensure nutritional adequacy.

- **Hydration**: Individuals with dysphagia are at risk of dehydration, especially if liquids are thickened. Ensuring adequate fluid intake is essential. Some may benefit from fluid-thickening agents prescribed by healthcare providers.

- **Caloric Needs**: Depending on the severity of dysphagia and individual factors like age and activity level, caloric needs may vary. Adjustments in portion sizes or frequency of meals may be necessary to meet energy requirements.

• **Nutrient Density**: Choosing nutrient-dense foods is important to maximize nutritional intake without increasing volume. This includes foods rich in vitamins, minerals, and protein.

• **Supplements**: In some cases, nutritional supplements (e.g., fortified drinks or vitamin/mineral supplements) may be recommended to address specific deficiencies or to ensure adequate nutrition.

• **Mealtime Environment**: Creating a supportive mealtime environment can improve eating experiences for individuals with dysphagia. This may include minimizing distractions, providing adequate time for meals, and using adaptive utensils if needed.

By addressing these considerations, healthcare providers and caregivers can help individuals with dysphagia maintain optimal nutrition and overall health.

Dysphagia Diet Levels

Dysphagia diets are often categorized into specific levels based on the texture and consistency of foods and liquids. Here are the commonly used diet levels:

Level 1: Pureed Foods

- Foods are smooth and cohesive with no lumps (e.g., pureed fruits, mashed potatoes, yogurt).
- Liquids are often thickened to nectar or pudding consistency.

Level 2: Mechanically Altered Foods

- Foods are moist and soft, requiring minimal chewing (e.g., soft cooked vegetables, ground meats, scrambled eggs).

- Liquids can be thicker but still pourable, like nectar consistency.

Level 3: Advanced (or Soft) Foods

- Foods are soft, and bite-sized pieces that can be chewed easily (e.g., tender meats, soft fruits, cooked pasta).
- Liquids are typically thin but may be modified for safety.

Level 4: Regular Diet (with precautions)

- Foods are regular texture but should be chewed thoroughly before swallowing (e.g., whole fruits, nuts, tough meats).

- Some individuals may require specific modifications or precautions when consuming these foods.

Additionally, liquids may be classified based on their viscosity, often using a thickening scale (thin, nectar-thick, honey-thick, or pudding-thick) to ensure safety during swallowing.

It's important to tailor these diet levels to individual needs, often in consultation with a healthcare provider or dietitian, based on the severity of dysphagia and swallowing abilities.

Texture Modification

Texture modification involves altering the consistency of foods and liquids to make them easier and safer to swallow for individuals with dysphagia. Here's a breakdown of common texture modifications:

• **Pureed Foods**: Foods are blended to a smooth, homogeneous consistency with no lumps. This includes items like applesauce, pureed meats, and smoothies.

• **Moist and Soft Foods**: Foods are cooked until soft and then cut into small, bite-sized pieces, making them easy to chew. Examples include soft vegetables, ground meats, and scrambled eggs.

• **Chopped or Minced Foods**: Foods are finely chopped or minced, allowing for easier chewing and swallowing. This may include finely chopped fruits, vegetables, or meats.

• **Thickened Liquids**: Liquids are modified to prevent aspiration and make swallowing easier. Common thickness levels include:

  • **Nectar-Thick**: Similar to the consistency of fruit nectar; pourable but thicker than water.

  • **Honey-Thick**: Similar to honey; flows slowly and drizzles off a spoon.

  • **Pudding-Thick**: Thick enough to hold its shape and not pourable.

• **Avoiding Certain Textures**: It's important to avoid foods that are hard, crunchy, sticky, or tough, as they can increase the risk of choking or aspiration.

Texture modification should be tailored to the individual's swallowing abilities and preferences, often determined by a speech-language pathologist or dietitian.

CHAPTER TWO
Meal Preparation And Cooking Techniques

Meal preparation and cooking techniques for individuals with dysphagia focus on making foods easier and safer to swallow. Here are some key methods:

• **Pureeing**: Use a blender or food processor to puree foods until smooth. Add liquids (like broth or milk) as needed to achieve the desired consistency.

• **Mashing**: For soft foods like potatoes or fruits, mashing can create a smooth texture without the need for pureeing. A fork or potato masher works well for this.

• **Steaming**: Steaming vegetables until soft preserves nutrients while making them easier to chew and swallow. Ensure they are well-cooked and tender.

- **Cooking Slowly**: Slow-cooking or braising meats can make them more tender and easier to chew. Consider using moist cooking methods to keep foods juicy.

- **Thickening Liquids**: Use commercial thickening agents to modify the consistency of liquids. Follow the manufacturer's instructions for the right proportions.

- **Chopping and Mincing**: Finely chop or mince foods like vegetables and meats to create bite-sized pieces that are easier to manage.

- **Avoiding Certain Cooking Methods**: Steer clear of frying or grilling tough meats, as they may become chewy and hard to swallow. Instead, opt for baking or steaming.

- **Adding Moisture**: Incorporate sauces, gravies, or broths to dry foods to enhance flavor and improve texture, making them easier to swallow.

By using these techniques, caregivers can prepare meals that meet the dietary needs of individuals with dysphagia while maintaining taste and variety.

Foods To Include And Avoid

Here's a guide on foods to include and avoid for individuals with dysphagia:

Foods to Include:

Pureed Foods:

- Applesauce
- Pureed vegetables (carrots, peas)
- Smooth yogurt or puddings
- Mashed potatoes

Moist and Soft Foods:

- Soft-cooked fruits (bananas, ripe pears)
- Scrambled or soft-boiled eggs
- Ground meats (with gravy or sauce)
- Soft fish (like salmon)

Thickened Liquids:

- Nectar-thick beverages (juice, smoothies)
- Honey-thick liquids (thickened soups, broths)
- Pudding-thick liquids (custards, thick shakes)

Tender Grains:

- Cooked oatmeal or cream of wheat
- Soft bread (without crusts)
- Cooked pasta (well-cooked, soft)

Foods to Avoid:

Hard or Crunchy Foods:

- Nuts and seeds
- Raw vegetables (carrots, celery)
- Hard candies and chips

Sticky or Tough Foods:

- Dried fruits (raisins, apricots)
- Tough cuts of meat (steak, jerky)
- Sticky foods (peanut butter)

Stringy or Fibrous Foods:

- Certain fruits (pineapple, oranges)
- Celery or other fibrous vegetables

Thin Liquids:

- Water
- Regular juice (unless thickened)
- Coffee or tea (unless thickened)

It's essential to tailor food choices based on individual swallowing abilities and preferences, often with the guidance of a healthcare provider or dietitian.

Breakfast Recipes

Here are some easy breakfast recipes suitable for individuals with dysphagia, focusing on texture modifications:

1. Pureed Oatmeal

Ingredients:

- 1/2 cup rolled oats
- 1 cup water or milk
- Sweetener (honey or sugar, optional)

Instructions:

- Cook oats in water or milk according to package instructions.
- Once cooked, blend until smooth. Add sweetener if desired.
- Serve warm. You can add pureed fruits for flavor.

2. Banana Pancakes:

Ingredients:

- 1 ripe banana
- 1 egg
- 1/4 cup oats (optional)

Instructions:

- Mash the banana in a bowl.
- Mix in the egg until well combined. If using oats, blend them into a fine flour and add.
- Cook on a non-stick skillet over low heat until golden on both sides.
- Serve warm, optionally with a thin layer of syrup or pureed fruit.

3. Smoothie Bowl:

Ingredients:

- 1 ripe banana
- 1/2 cup yogurt (plain or flavored)
- 1/2 cup soft fruit (berries, peaches)
- 1/4 cup milk or juice

Instructions:

- Blend all ingredients until smooth.
- Pour into a bowl. You can top it with a thin layer of pureed fruit for added flavor.

4. Scrambled Eggs with Cheese:

Ingredients:

- 2 eggs
- 1 tablespoon milk

- Soft cheese (like cream cheese or cheddar, finely shredded)

Instructions:

- Whisk eggs and milk together in a bowl.
- Cook in a non-stick skillet over low heat, stirring gently.
- Once eggs are nearly set, add cheese and continue to cook until melted and creamy.
- Serve warm.

5. Apple Sauce Muffins:

Ingredients:

- 1 cup unsweetened applesauce
- 1 cup flour (whole wheat or all-purpose)
- 1/2 teaspoon baking powder
- 1/2 teaspoon cinnamon (optional)

Instructions:

- Preheat the oven to 350°F (175°C) and line a muffin tin with liners.
- Mix all ingredients in a bowl until combined.
- Pour batter into muffin tins and bake for 15-20 minutes or until a toothpick comes out clean.
- Allow to cool before serving.

These recipes are easy to modify further based on individual preferences and dietary needs.

Lunch Recipes

Here are some easy lunch recipes suitable for individuals with dysphagia, focusing on texture modifications:

1. Creamy Tomato Soup:

Ingredients:

- 1 can (14 oz) crushed tomatoes
- 1 cup vegetable or chicken broth
- 1/2 cup cream or milk
- Salt and pepper to taste
- Fresh basil (optional)

Instructions:

- In a saucepan, combine crushed tomatoes and broth. Heat over medium until warm.
- Use an immersion blender to blend until smooth.

- Stir in cream and season with salt and pepper. Heat gently.
- Serve warm, garnished with fresh basil if desired.

2. Mashed Sweet Potatoes:

Ingredients:

- 2 medium sweet potatoes
- 1 tablespoon butter or margarine
- 1/4 cup milk
- Salt and cinnamon (optional)

Instructions:

- Peel and chop sweet potatoes. Boil in water until tender (about 15-20 minutes).
- Drain and mash with butter and milk until smooth. Add salt and cinnamon to taste.
- Serve warm.

3. Smooth Chicken Salad:

Ingredients:

- 1 cup cooked chicken (shredded or diced)
- 1/4 cup mayonnaise
- 1 tablespoon yogurt (optional)
- Soft fruits (like mashed avocado or pureed apples)

Instructions:

- In a bowl, mix cooked chicken with mayonnaise and yogurt until well combined.
- If desired, mix in mashed avocado or pureed apples for added creaminess.
- Serve on soft bread or alone.

4. Pureed Vegetable Medley:

Ingredients:

- 1 cup mixed vegetables (carrots, peas, spinach)
- 1 cup vegetable broth
- Salt and pepper to taste

Instructions:

- Steam or boil the mixed vegetables until tender.
- Blend with vegetable broth until smooth. Adjust consistency with more broth if needed.
- Season with salt and pepper before serving.

5. Soft Cheese and Avocado Wrap:

Ingredients:

- 1 soft tortilla or flatbread

- 1/4 cup cream cheese or soft cheese
- 1/2 ripe avocado (mashed)

Instructions:

- Spread cream cheese evenly on the tortilla.
- Add mashed avocado and roll the tortilla tightly.
- Slice into bite-sized pieces for easier consumption.

These recipes can be tailored to suit individual tastes and dietary needs, ensuring they are both nutritious and enjoyable.

Here are some easy dinner recipes suitable for individuals with dysphagia, focusing on texture modifications:

1. Creamy Chicken and Rice Casserole:

Ingredients:

- 1 cup cooked chicken (shredded)
- 1 cup cooked rice
- 1 cup cream of chicken soup (or homemade)
- 1/2 cup milk
- Soft vegetables (like peas or carrots)

Instructions:

- Preheat oven to 350°F (175°C).
- In a mixing bowl, combine shredded chicken, cooked rice,

cream of chicken soup, milk, and soft vegetables.

- Transfer to a greased baking dish and spread evenly.
- Bake for 25-30 minutes or until heated through. Serve warm.

2. Pureed Spinach and Ricotta Pasta:

Ingredients:

- 1 cup cooked pasta (soft, like macaroni or small shells)
- 1 cup fresh spinach (cooked until wilted)
- 1/2 cup ricotta cheese
- 1/4 cup milk
- Salt and pepper to taste

Instructions:

- In a blender, combine cooked pasta, wilted spinach, ricotta cheese, and milk. Blend until smooth.

- If the mixture is too thick, add more milk to reach desired consistency.
- Serve warm, seasoned with salt and pepper.

3. Soft Beef Stew:

Ingredients:

- 1 lb beef (cut into small cubes)
- 2 cups soft vegetables (carrots, potatoes, peas)
- 4 cups beef broth
- Salt and pepper to taste
- Optional: herbs like thyme or bay leaf

Instructions:

- In a pot, brown beef cubes in a little oil.
- Add broth and vegetables. Bring to a boil, then reduce heat to simmer.
- Cook for about 1.5 hours, or until beef is tender. Blend if needed for a smoother consistency.
- Serve warm.

4. Egg and Spinach Muffins:

Ingredients:

- 4 eggs
- 1/2 cup milk
- 1 cup cooked spinach (chopped)
- 1/4 cup cheese (shredded, optional)
- Salt and pepper to taste

Instructions:

- Preheat oven to 350°F (175°C) and grease a muffin tin.
- In a bowl, whisk together eggs and milk. Stir in chopped spinach and cheese.
- Pour the mixture into muffin cups, filling them about halfway.
- Bake for 15-20 minutes or until set. Allow to cool slightly before serving.

5. Soft Fish with Lemon Sauce:

Ingredients:

- 2 fillets of soft fish (like tilapia or cod)
- 1 tablespoon lemon juice
- 1 tablespoon butter
- Salt and pepper to taste

Instructions:

- Preheat oven to 375°F (190°C).
- Place fish fillets in a baking dish. Drizzle with lemon juice and dot with butter. Season with salt and pepper.
- Bake for 15-20 minutes, or until fish flakes easily with a fork.
- Serve warm, optionally with pureed vegetables on the side.

These recipes can be adjusted to suit individual preferences and dietary restrictions, ensuring a nutritious and enjoyable meal.

CHAPTER THREE
Snack Ideas For Dysphagia Patients

Here are some snack ideas suitable for individuals with dysphagia, focusing on texture modifications:

1. Applesauce Cups:

• Store-bought or homemade applesauce is easy to swallow and comes in various flavors.

2. Smoothies:

• Blend soft fruits (like bananas, berries, or peaches) with yogurt or milk for a nutritious, drinkable snack. You can adjust thickness with added liquid.

3. Pureed Hummus:

• Serve pureed hummus with soft, well-cooked vegetables (like carrots or zucchini) for dipping. You can also use soft pita bread or crackers.

4. Greek Yogurt:

• Plain or flavored Greek yogurt is creamy and can be topped with pureed fruits or a drizzle of honey.

5. Cheese Spread:

• Soft cheese spreads (like cream cheese or ricotta) can be enjoyed on soft bread or crackers.

6. Pudding or Custard:

• Ready-made or homemade pudding and custard provide a sweet, smooth option that is easy to swallow.

7. Mashed Avocado:

• Serve mashed avocado on soft bread or alone, seasoned with a bit of salt and lemon juice for flavor.

8. Pureed Soups:

• Small servings of pureed soups (like butternut squash or tomato) can be enjoyed warm as a snack.

9. Soft Banana or Pear:

• Ripe bananas or peeled, ripe pears can be mashed or sliced into small, manageable pieces.

10. Rice Pudding:

• A soft, sweet option that is creamy and easy to swallow, perfect for a light snack.

These snacks can be tailored to individual tastes and preferences while ensuring safety and enjoyment.

Managing Social Aspects Of Eating

Managing the social aspects of eating for individuals with dysphagia can enhance their dining experiences and overall quality of life. Here are some strategies to consider:

1. Communication:

• **Informing Others**: Share dietary needs and swallowing difficulties with family and friends to foster understanding and support.

• **Express Preferences**: Encourage the individual to express their food preferences and comfort levels when dining out or at gatherings.

2. Creating a Supportive Environment:

• **Choose Comfortable Settings**: Opt for quiet, relaxed dining environments to reduce distractions and stress during meals.

• **Seating Arrangements**: Ensure the individual is seated comfortably and can easily access food and drinks.

3. Meal Planning:

• **Involve in Planning**: Encourage participation in meal planning and preparation to maintain interest and control over food choices.

• **Consider Texture Modifications**: When planning meals with others, discuss texture modifications to ensure safety and enjoyment.

<u>4. **Social Inclusion**</u>:

•   **Join   Group   Meals**: Encourage participation in group meals, focusing on social interaction rather than just food.

• **Host Inclusive Gatherings**: Host meals where the menu accommodates all guests, including those with dysphagia.

5. Adapted Utensils and Tools:

• **Use Appropriate Utensils**: Consider using adaptive utensils designed for easier handling and safer eating.

• **Encourage Self-Feeding**: Whenever possible, allow the individual to feed themselves, promoting independence.

6. Focus on Enjoyment:

• **Emphasize the Social Experience**: Encourage conversations and interactions during meals to shift focus away from food alone.

• **Celebrate Food**: Consider making mealtime special with themed meals, favorite dishes, or festive occasions.

7. Educate Others:

• **Provide Information**: Share information about dysphagia with friends and family to promote understanding and reduce stigma.

• **Cooking Together**: Engage family members or friends in cooking together, making it a fun and collaborative experience.

By fostering a supportive and inclusive atmosphere around meals, individuals with dysphagia can enjoy the social aspects of eating while managing their dietary needs effectively.

Monitoring And Adjusting The Diet

Monitoring and adjusting the diet for individuals with dysphagia is crucial for ensuring safety and nutritional adequacy. Here are some key steps to consider:

1. Regular Assessment:

• **Swallowing Evaluations**: Periodically reassess swallowing abilities through clinical evaluations or swallow studies (like MBSS or FEES) to identify any changes.

• **Nutritional Status**: Monitor weight and overall nutritional status, looking for signs of malnutrition or dehydration.

2. Track Symptoms:

• **Document Difficulties**: Keep a log of any swallowing difficulties, such as coughing, choking, or discomfort, to identify patterns and triggers.

• **Feedback on Foods**: Note which foods are easier or harder to swallow and any adverse reactions.

3. Adjust Textures:

• **Modify Food Consistency**: Based on assessments, adjust food textures as needed (e.g., move from pureed to minced if swallowing improves).

- **Thicken Liquids**: Regularly check the viscosity of liquids and adjust thickness based on individual tolerance.

4. Consult Healthcare Professionals:

- **Dietitian Involvement**: Work with a registered dietitian specializing in dysphagia to tailor dietary plans and ensure nutritional needs are met.

- **Speech-Language Pathologist**: Collaborate with a speech-language pathologist for ongoing swallowing therapy and support.

5. Adapt to Changes:

- **Monitor Health Conditions**: Changes in health status (e.g., illness, medication changes) may necessitate dietary adjustments.

• **Be Responsive**: Be willing to change foods and textures as needed based on comfort and safety levels.

6. Incorporate Preferences:

• **Personal Preferences**: Include the individual's food preferences in meal planning to enhance enjoyment and compliance with dietary recommendations.

• **Variety**: Ensure a variety of foods to provide balanced nutrition and prevent monotony.

7. Education:

• **Teach Caregivers and Family**: Educate those involved in meal preparation and feeding about dysphagia and dietary modifications to ensure consistency and safety.

By actively monitoring and adjusting the diet, caregivers can help individuals with dysphagia maintain optimal nutrition while minimizing risks associated with swallowing difficulties.

CHAPTER FOUR
Coping Strategies For Patients And Caregivers

Coping strategies for patients with dysphagia and their caregivers can help manage the challenges associated with this condition. Here are some effective strategies:

For Patients:

- **Education**: Learn about dysphagia, dietary modifications, and safe swallowing techniques to feel empowered and informed.

- **Focus on Enjoyment**: Shift attention from difficulties to the social aspects of eating, emphasizing enjoyment and connection during meals.

- **Mindful Eating**: Practice mindfulness during meals, focusing on each bite and chewing thoroughly to improve swallowing safety.

- **Experiment with Textures**: Explore different textures and flavors within dietary guidelines to find enjoyable options.

- **Use Adaptive Tools**: Consider using specialized utensils or cups designed for easier handling and safer eating.

For Caregivers:

- **Educate Yourself**: Understand dysphagia and its implications to provide informed support and make appropriate dietary choices.

- **Encourage Communication**: Foster open communication with the individual about their preferences and any discomfort they may experience.

- **Meal Preparation Together**: Involve the individual in meal planning and preparation to enhance their sense of control and engagement.

- **Create a Supportive Environment**: Ensure a calm and comfortable dining atmosphere, free from distractions, to promote relaxation during meals.

- **Practice Patience**: Be patient and supportive during mealtimes, allowing extra time for eating and encouraging independence where possible.

Shared Strategies:

- **Seek Support Groups**: Join support groups or communities for individuals with dysphagia and their caregivers to share experiences and resources.

- **Regular Check-ins**: Have regular discussions about dietary needs, preferences, and any emerging challenges, fostering a team approach to care.

- **Self-Care**: Caregivers should prioritize self-care, recognizing their own needs and seeking support when needed to prevent burnout.

These strategies can be implemented to more effectively address the challenges of dysphagia, thereby improving the quality of life and promoting a positive dining experience for both patients and caregivers.

Conclusion

The management of dysphagia necessitates a comprehensive approach that encompasses the comprehension of the condition, the implementation of dietary modifications, and the encouragement of social interactions during meals.

The eating experience can be improved for both patients and caregivers by concentrating on safe swallowing practices, monitoring nutritional intake, and adapting to individual requirements. In order to establish a supportive environment, it is imperative to engage in effective communication, education, and collaboration with healthcare professionals.

Individuals with dysphagia can enhance their quality of life, maintain nutritional health, and appreciate mealtimes with the utilization of appropriate strategies and resources.

THE END